THE SURGICAL ONCOLOGY REVIEW

For the **ABSITE** and **Boards**

A R Y A N   M E K N A T ,   M . D .

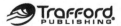

www.trafford.com
North America & international
toll-free: 844-688-6899 (USA & Canada)
fax: 812 355 4082

CONTENTS

CONTRIBUTORS

Aaron Blackham, MD, FACS, FSSO
Division of Surgical Oncology
Lehigh Valley Health Network
Allentown, Pennsylvania

Heiwon Chung, MD
Division of Surgical Oncology
Lehigh Valley Health Network
Allentown, Pennsylvania

Lori Alfonse, DO, FACOS, MEng
Division of Surgical Oncology
Medical Director, Lehigh Valley Health Network Breast
Health Services
Allentown, Pennsylvania

Aaron Jacobs, MD
Resident, Department of Plastic Surgery
Lehigh Valley Health Network
Allentown, Pennsylvania

Jeffrey Brodsky, MD
Division of Surgical Oncology
Lehigh Valley Health Network
Allentown, Pennsylvania

DEDICATIONS

To Dr. Kothuru – who saw potential in me and taught me to have respect and reverence for the power that knowledge yields.

To Dr. Relles – who is the embodiment of compassion and empathy, and from whom I learned that being an educator is more about creating the right environment for learning rather than just the delivery of information.

To my family – Mahsa, Denna, and Mina – thank you for your never-ending support and being my living reminder of what's most important in life.

PREFACE

Surgical oncology, in the context of general surgery, is very high yield for exams and in clinical practice. General surgeons are required to know how to screen, workup, and treat a wide spectrum of malignancies. As it stands now, there are no review books dedicated to the topic of surgical oncology, which can account for a fair amount of the general surgery inservice and board exams.

This material is not all encompassing but designed to have the reader prepared for surgical oncology questions that can come up on the ABSITE, American Board of Surgery Qualifying and Certifying Exam. Using this material alone will not guarantee a passing score on the boards, nor is this review intended to be utilized as a substitute for clinical competency.

This material is a culmination of the notes I have organized over my five years of general surgery residency. I was motivated to create a concise review dedicated to surgical oncology, given that the material is often glossed over in other review books or often buried in the middle or end of long textbook chapters. The most commonly encountered questions are "best next step" questions, which can be difficult if there's no foundational knowledge of the pathology at hand. This format is designed to have a systematic and algorithmic approach to various cancers. This outline format includes

- General overview
- Screening guidelines, if applicable
- Diagnosis
- Staging, if applicable
- Tumor markers, if applicable
  o Associated gene mutation(s)

- Therapy
  o Surgical
  o Neo- and/or adjuvant therapy, if applicable
- Follow-up

Although this review has been specifically geared for general surgery residents taking the ABSITE, the information within *The Surgical Oncology Review* could be utilized by other groups:

- General surgery residents preparing for the American Board of Surgery Qualifying and Certifying Exam
- Board certified general surgeons looking to review for their American Board of Surgery recertification examination
- Medical students — they can use this resource as a guide while rotating through a general surgery or surgical oncology service
- Advanced practice clinicians (i.e., advance practice nurse practitioners and physician assistants) — while working with general surgeons or surgical oncologists

MELANOMA

General Overview

- The most lethal skin cancer – representing only 1% of skin cancers but accounting for over 80% of skin cancer deaths
- Risk factors:
  - Congenital nevi – 10% lifetime risk
  - Familial BK mole syndrome (**CPKN2A mutation**) – 100% risk of melanoma
  - Xeroderma pigmentosa (**autosomal recessive, unable to repair damaged DNA after UV damage**)
- Prognosis worse for:
  - Men
  - Ulcerated lesions
  - Ocular and mucosal lesions
- Lung is most common location for distant melanoma metastases but can metastasize to almost any site, including liver, brain, non-regional lymph nodes, bones, skin, GI tract
- Melanoma is the most common primary source of metastatic small bowel lesions
- Types:
  - **Melanoma in situ or thin lentigo maligna** (Hutchinson's freckle) – confined to the epidermis. No potential for metastases, need wide local excision with negative margins
  - **Lentigo maligna melanoma** – least aggressive, minimal invasion, radial growth pattern first, seen in elderly patients
  - **Superficial spreading** – most common type, intermediate malignancy risk, often found on the trunk or upper extremities, evolves from nevus or sun-exposed areas

- o **Acral lentiginous** – very aggressive, found on the palms and/or soles of African Americans, can be subungual
- o **Nodular** – most aggressive type, most likely to have metastasized at time of diagnosis, vertical growth pattern first, can occur anywhere on the body
- o Treatment is not determined by specific subtype

Screening

- Physical exam, head to toe – for high-risk patients
- Signs of melanoma (**ABCDE**)
  - o A – asymmetry (angulations, indentation, notching, ulceration, bleeding)
  - o B – borders that are irregular
  - o C – color changes (darkening)
    - 1-2% of melanomas are non-pigmented
  - o D – diameter (>/= 8 mm)
  - o E – elevation or evolving over time
    - All the above are highly sensitive but not specific
- Blue color – ominous sign

Diagnosis/Staging

- *Diagnosis*
  - o "Suspicious pigmented lesions" should undergo a **shave** or **punch biopsy**
    - If the lesion comes back as melanoma, the pathologist should comment on:
      - Breslow depth
      - Mitotic rate
      - Ulceration
      - Deep and peripheral margin status
    - No difference in outcome between shave and punch biopsy

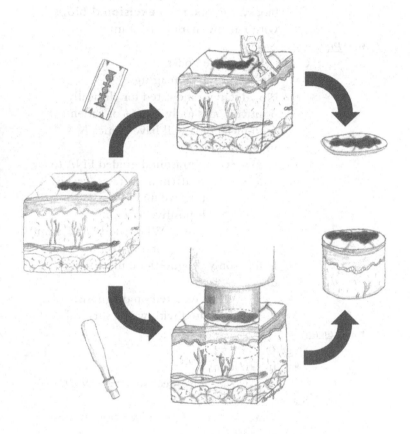

- **Shave biopsy** – diagnosis easier to obtain (obtained from interface between normal skin and lesion)
- **Punch biopsy** – less likely to have an inaccurate deep margin
- If lesions are too large for shave or punch biopsy, can obtain an **excisional biopsy** with narrow margins (1–4 mm)

- *Preoperative Staging*
  - Clinically negative nodes
    - No preoperative imaging
    - Nodal staging indicated for clinically positive nodes (only 5–10% of patients with melanoma will have clinically involved nodes)
      - Ultrasound guided FNA to confirm metastases (versus reactive nodes)
      - If positive, obtain
        - Whole body PET scan
        - Brain MRI
    - LDH – only prognostic in metastatic disease
      - When elevated on diagnosis, associated with worse survival

- *Staging*
  - Stage 0
    - In situ lesions
      - Five-year survival – 99.9%
  - Stage 1
    - T1a – $\leq$ 1 mm, no ulceration, mitosis < 1 mm^2
    - T1b – $\leq$ 1 mm, with ulceration, mitosis > 1 mm^2
    - T2a – 1–2 mm, no ulceration, mitosis < 1 mm^2
      - Five-year survival – 89–95%

- o Stage 2
  - T2b – 1–2 mm, with ulceration, mitosis > 1 mm^2
  - T3a – 2–4 mm, no ulceration, mitosis < 1 mm^2
  - T3b – 2–4 mm, with ulceration, mitosis > 1 mm^2
  - T4a – > 4 mm, no ulceration, mitosis < 1 mm^2
  - T4b – > 4 mm, with ulceration, mitosis > 1 mm^2
    - o Five-year survival – 45–79%
- o Stage 3
  - N1 – single positive lymph node
    - N1a – micrometastasis
    - N1b – macrometastasis
  - N2 – two to three positive lymph nodes or regional in-transit
    - N2a – micrometastasis
    - N2b – macrometastasis
    - N2c – in-transit metastasis/satellite lesions *without* metastatic nodes
  - N3 – four positive lymph nodes, matted nodes, in-transit metastasis/satellite lesions *with* metastatic nodes
    - o Five-year survival – 24–70%
- o Stage 4
  - M1a – metastases to the skin, subcutaneous tissue, or distant lymph nodes
    - Normal LDH
  - M1b – metastases to the lungs
    - Normal LDH
  - M1c – other visceral metastases
    - Elevated LDH
      - o Five-year survival – 7–19%

Tumor Markers

- *Associated Gene Mutations*
    o **BRAF V600E** – seen in 50% of melanomas
    o MAPK signaling pathway
    o NRAS
    o KIT
    o PTEN

Therapy

- Wide local excision – recommended surgical margins for excision based on Breslow thickness
    o In situ – 0.5 cm
    o Thin (</= 1 mm) – 1 cm
    o Thick > 1 mm – 2 cm
        ▪ Depth of excision should be down to muscle fascia
- Perform **sentinel lymph node biopsy** if:
    o Nodes clinically negative
    o Breslow thickness >/= 0.8 mm
    o Ulcerated lesions
        ▪ MSLT – II Trial
            • Patients with positive SLNBx randomized to completion lymphadenectomy versus US surveillance (every four months for two years then every six months every three years).
            • Main outcomes:
                o No difference in melanoma-specific survival between the two groups
                o Higher regional failure in US surveillance group (in general, patients went on to have lymph node dissection)

- o Higher rates of lymphedema in the lymphadenectomy group
  - US surveillance is now standard of care which avoids the morbidity of non-therapeutic lymph node dissection with equivalent survival.
- **Superficial Parotidectomy** – for all scalp/face melanomas anterior to the ear and above the lip >/= 1 mm in depth, including melanomas on the ear
- **Complete node dissection** is indicated when patient present with clinically positive lymph nodes (e.g., stations 1–3 in axilla)

Neo- and Adjuvant Therapy

- No effective chemotherapy for melanoma
- Interferon and IL-2 indicated in the past but no longer used
- Immunotherapy (PD1 and CTLA inhibitors) and Targeted Therapies (BRAF and MEK inhibitors) are effective in the metastatic setting and beneficial as adjuvant treatment in patients with:
  - o Node positive (Stage 3) and high-risk Stage 2B patients
  - o These treatments are also being used increasingly in the neoadjuvant setting in patients who present with bulky Stage 3 or resectable Stage 4 disease
    - **Vemurafenib** or **Dabrafenib** – for BRAF (+) mutation associated Melanomas
    - **Trametinimb** or **Cobimetinib** – MEK inhibitors, used with BRAF inhibitors
    - **Pembrolizumab** – blockade of PD 1 – PD L2 interactions
    - **Ipilimumab** – blockade of CTLA – four pathways

Follow-up

- History and physical exam
  - o Every three to six months for three years, then every four to twelve months for two years, then annually thereafter
- CT surveillance every six to twelve months for five years for patients with Stage 3

NOTES

HEAD AND NECK CANCER

General Overview

Squamous cell carcinoma – the most common head and neck cancer
- Risk Factors:
  - o Alcohol
  - o Tobacco products
    - Both of which have a synergistic effect
  - o HPV
- Subsites:
  - o Oral Cavity
  - o Pharynx
    - Nasopharynx
    - Oropharynx
    - Hypopharynx
  - o Larynx
  - o Salivary glands
- **Modified radical neck dissection (MRND)**
  - o Take omohyoid, submandibular gland, sensory nerves C2-C5, cervical branch of facial nerve, ipsilateral thyroid lobe, lymph node stations 2–5
- **Radical neck dissection (RND)**
  - o Same MRND *plus* take CN XI (accessory nerve), ipsilateral SCM, and ipsilateral IJ

Diagnosis/Staging

- *Diagnosis*
  - o Workup of an asymptomatic head and neck mass
    - H&P
    - Laryngoscopy
    - FNA
    - Panendoscopy (laryngoscopy, upper endoscopy, and bronchoscopy)
    - CT of neck and chest

- Excisional biopsy if FNA is unrevealing, with re-excision for margins if cancer
  - Preauricular masses are parotid tumors until proven otherwise
    - Dx: **Superficial parotidectomy** – for tissue diagnosis
  - If neck mass is a positive lymph node, without a known primary
    - Panendoscopy (with random biopsies)
    - CT scan neck/chest/abdomen/pelvis
    - If still can't find primary
      - Ipsilateral MRND, ipsilateral tonsillectomy, bilateral neck radiation
      - **Tonsils** – most common location for occult head and neck malignancies
- *Staging*
  - Each subsite has its own staging system and treatment recommendations
  - In general (for the purposes of the ABSITE and ABS Qualifying exam):
    - Stages 1 and 2 – local disease (no regional or distant metastases)
    - Stages 3 and 4 – either locally aggressive or distant metastases
    - Treatment for Stages 1 and 2 is either surgery or radiation, depending on subsite
    - Treatment for Stages 3 and 4 is multimodal – surgery followed by radiation +/- chemotherapy

Therapy

- *Oral Cavity Cancer*
  - Lower lip – most common site
  - Treatment:

- Wide resection with 1 cm margins for tumors:
  - < 4 cm
  - No nodal or bony invasion
- Wide resection with 1 cm margins, MRND, and XRT for tumors:
  - >/= 4 cm
  - Clinically positive lymph nodes
  - Bony invasion
- *Nasopharyngeal Cancer*
  - Associated with EBV
  - Spreads to posterior cervical lymph nodes
    - The most common presentation is painless neck mass
  - Treatment:
    - XRT primary therapy (very radio-sensitive)
    - Chemo-XRT for advanced disease (no role for surgery)
- *Oropharyngeal Cancer*
  - Spreads to posterior cervical lymph nodes
  - Treatment:
    - XRT for tumors:
      - < 4 cm
      - No nodal or bony invasion
    - Wide resection with 1 cm margins, MRND, and XRT for tumors:
      - >/= 4 cm
      - Clinically positive lymph nodes
      - Bony invasion
- *Hypopharyngeal Cancer*
  - Spreads to anterior cervical lymph nodes
  - Treatment:
    - XRT for tumors:
      - < 4 cm
      - No nodal or bony invasion

- Wide resection with 1 cm margins, MRND, and XRT for tumors:
  - $>/= 4$ cm
- _Laryngeal Cancer_
  - o Treatment:
    - XRT if only the vocal cords are involved
    - Chemo-XRT if beyond vocal cords
    - Resection with XRT if vocal cords are fixed
      - MRND if there is nodal invasion
- _Salivary Gland Cancers_
  - o Mass in large salivary gland – more likely to be benign
  - o Mass in small salivary gland – more likely to be malignant, although parotid gland is the most frequent site for malignant tumors
    - **Mucoepidermoid CA**
      - No. 1 malignant tumor of the salivary glands
    - **Adenoid cystic CA**
      - No. 2 malignant tumor of the salivary glands
      - Long indolent course
      - Propensity to invade nerve roots
      - Very radiosensitive
    - Treatment for both:
      - Resection of gland (e.g., total parotidectomy), prophylactic MRND, and post-operative XRT
        - o For _low-grade malignant_ parotid gland tumors: Superficial parotidectomy with XRT
        - o For _benign_ parotid gland tumors: Superficial parotidectomy

- Most common injured nerve with parotidectomy – **greater auricular nerve** (numbness overlying lower ear)
- Most common injured nerve with submandibular gland resection – **marginal mandibular nerve** (commissure droop, corner of mouth)

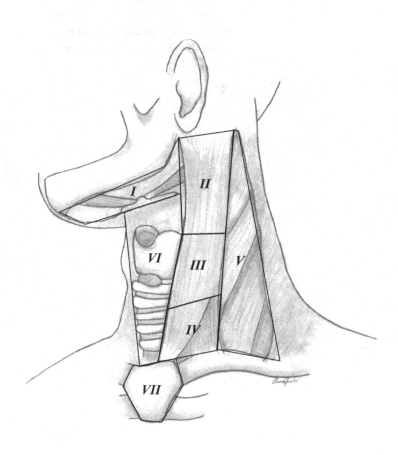

NOTES

BREAST CANCER

General Overview

- US breast cancer risk – one in eight women (12%)
- Screening decreases mortality by 25%
- Clinical features
  - Distortion of normal architecture
  - Skin/nipple distortion or retraction
  - Hard
  - Tethered
  - Indistinct borders
- **Bone** – most common site for distant metastasis (via Batson's venous plexus)

Screening

- **Screening mammography** (there's a difference between screening and diagnostic mammography)
  - 90% sensitivity/specificity
  - Less sensitive with dense breast tissue (younger patients)
  - Findings suggestive of cancer
    - Irregular borders, spiculated, calcifications, ductal asymmetry, distortion of architecture
- Screening guidelines:
  - *Low-risk patients*
    - Every two to three years starting at age 40
    - Annually after age 50
  - *High-risk patients* (BRCA 1 and 2, Li-Fraumeni, Cowden syndrome, Peutz-Jeghers, ATM, CHEK2, CDH1)
    - Ten years before youngest age of diagnosis in first-degree relative
    - Annual screening mammogram and MRI starting at age 25

- For BRCA 1 and 2 patients
- **BI-RADS Classification** (based on *diagnostic mammography*)
  - o **0**, not enough info (screening mammogram) – further imaging (diagnostic mammogram)
  - o **1**, negative – routine follow-up
  - o **2**, benign – routine follow-up
  - o **3**, probably benign – short interval follow-up (six months)
  - o **4**, suspicious for malignancy – core needle biopsy
  - o **5**, highly suggestive for malignancy – core needle biopsy
  - o **6**, biopsy confirmed malignancy - excision

Diagnosis/Staging

- *Diagnosis*
  - o Symptomatic breast mass workup
    - ▪ < 40 years old
      - Ultrasound
      - Core needle biopsy
      - Need mammogram (unilateral) if clinical exam or ultrasound is indeterminate
    - ▪ > 40 years old
      - Need bilateral mammogram
      - Ultrasound
      - Core needle biopsy
  - o **Core needle biopsy** – provides architecture and pathology
  - o **FNA** – provides cytology (for lymph nodes)
  - o **Stereotactic needle biopsy**
    - ▪ For non-palpable lesions, mammographically guided CNBx
  - o Indications for *excisional biopsy* after core needle biopsy
    - ▪ Atypical ductal hyperplasia

- Atypical lobular hyperplasia
- Radial scar
- LCIS – pleomorphic LICS is a more aggressive subtype that is difficult to differ from DCIS and associated with infiltrating pleomorphic lobular carcinoma (requires negative margins)
- Papillary lesions with atypia
- Phyllodes tumor
- **Lack of concordance** between appearance of mammographic lesion and histologic diagnosis
- Nondiagnostic specimen

- _Staging_
  - TNM
    - T0 – no evidence of primary tumor
    - Tis – carcinoma in situ, Paget's disease of the nipple with no underlying tumor
    - T1 – < 2 cm
    - T2 – 2–5 cm
    - T3 – > 5 cm
    - T4 – any size with direct extension to the chest wall, skin edema, skin ulceration, satellite skin nodules, or inflammatory carcinoma
      - N0 – no regional node metastases
      - N1 – one to three ipsilateral axillary nodes, or an internal mammary (IM) node with microscopic disease
      - N2 – four to nine ipsilateral axillary nodes, or a clinically apparent IM node, matted/fixed nodes
      - N3 – ten or more ipsilateral axillary nodes, infraclavicular nodes, IM nodes in the presence

of axillary lymphadenopathy, or supraclavicular nodes
- o M0 – no metastases
- o M1 – distant metastases, or positive contralateral axillary nodes

- o **Stage grouping**
  - One of the few cancers where you do need to know the staging well
  - The way I remember them:
    - Stage 1 – **T1**
    - Stage 2a – T1, N1 or T2, N0
    - Stage 2b – T2, N1 or T3, N0
    - Stage 3a – **everything in between**
    - Stage 3b – **T4**, N-any
    - Stage 3c – T-any, **N3**
    - Stage 4 – **M1**

Tumor Markers

- *Associated Gene Mutations (not tumor markers)*
  - o Li-Fraumeni – *p53 mutation*
  - o Cowden syndrome – *PTEN*
  - o Peutz-Jeghers – *STK11*
  - o *CDH1*
  - o **BRCA 1**
    - Autosomal dominant
    - Chromosome 17
    - Triple negative and poorly differentiated tumors
      - 60% lifetime risk of female breast cancer
      - 40% lifetime risk of ovarian cancer
      - 1% lifetime risk of male breast cancer

- o **BRCA 2**
  - Autosomal dominant
  - Chromosome 15
  - Hormone receptor positive and well-differentiated tumors
    - 60% lifetime risk of female breast cancer
    - 10% lifetime risk of ovarian cancer
    - 10% lifetime risk of male breast cancer
    - Increased risk of prostate and pancreatic cancer

Therapy

- **Contraindications to Breast Conservation Therapy (BCT)**
  - o Absolute contraindications
    - Multicentric disease – two or more primary tumors in separate quadrants
    - Persistent positive margins
    - History of prior therapeutic irradiation, given need for adjuvant radiation, resulting in excessively high radiation dose
    - Diffuse malignant-appearing calcifications
    - Inflammatory breast cancer
  - o Relative contraindications
    - >/= T3 lesions
    - A history of scleroderma or active SLE
    - Large tumor in small breast that would result in unacceptable cosmesis
- For patients without contraindications, BCT entails:
  - o *Lumpectomy, sentinel lymph node biopsy, adjuvant radiation to ipsilateral chest wall and axilla (only radiate axilla if lymph nodes are involved)*

- Margins – "no ink on tumor"
  - For DCIS and pleomorphic LCIS – 2 mm margins (given radial growth pattern)
- BCT and simple mastectomy have similar oncologic outcomes with equivalent overall survival rates
- <u>ACOSOG Z-11 Trial</u>
  - Axillary lymph node dissection does not improve survival or local control compared to nodal observation in patients with T1-2 breast cancer and a positive sentinel lymph node biopsy (< 3 positive SLN) undergoing lumpectomy and whole-breast radiation
- For patients with contraindications:
  - *Modified radical mastectomy (MRM)*
    - Removes all breast tissue, including the nipple areolar complex
    - Includes axillary node dissection (level 1 and 2 nodes)

Neo- and Adjuvant Therapy

- **Neoadjuvant Therapy**
  - Indications for *neoadjuvant chemotherapy*
    - (+) HER-2 neu receptor
    - (-) Estrogen/Progesterone receptors
    - (+) Lymphadenopathy
    - (+) Oncotype Dx
    - Inflammatory breast cancer
  - Taxanes, Adriamycin, and Cyclophosphamide (TAC) for six to twelve weeks
  - *Trastuzumab* (Herceptin)
    - Given in the neoadjuvant setting – for (+) HER-2 neu receptors

- Monoclonal antibody
- Decreases risk of breast cancer recurrence by 50%
- Side effects – cardiac disease (heart failure, MI)
- **Adjuvant Therapy**
  - *Radiotherapy* (XRT)
    - Usually consists of 5,000 rad
    - Indicated after:
      - BCT
      - After MRM with:
        - >/= T3
        - >/= N2
        - Positive margins
        - Inflammatory breast cancer
    - Decreases rate of local recurrence
    - Women > 70 years old having a BCT or T1 disease can avoid XRT
      - ONLY IF they are ER/PR positive and have clinically negative nodes
  - *Tamoxifen*
    - Decreases risk of breast cancer recurrence by 50%
    - Blocks estrogen and progesterone receptors
    - Given in the adjuvant setting
    - Side effects – 1% risk of blood clots, 0.1% risk of endometrial cancer
    - Decreases risk of osteoporosis and fractures
  - *Aromatase inhibitors* (Anastrozole)
    - Only to be used for post-menopausal women
    - Block conversion of testosterone to estrogen in the periphery
    - Side effects – fractures
    - Decreased risk of thromboembolic events and endometrial cancer compared to tamoxifen

NOTES

PARATHYROID CANCER

General Overview

- Rare cause of hypercalcemia
- Compared with patients with a parathyroid adenoma, parathyroid carcinomas are more likely to present with
  - Neck mass
  - Bone and kidney disease
  - Marked hypercalcemia
  - Very high serum PTH levels
- Lung parenchyma is the most common location for metastases
- Mortality is due to complications from hypercalcemia
- Factors associated with reduced survival:
  - Males
  - Older age at diagnosis
  - Presence of metastases
- 50% five-year survival

Diagnosis

- Elevated calcium level
  - Generally, have very high calcium levels ($>/= 15$)
  - May have an associated palpable mass
- Elevated PTH
- Elevated alkaline phosphatase (ALP)
- Localization
  - Ultrasound
  - Sestamibi/SPECT scan (single photon emission CT)
  - The main role for CT and MRI is to assess for metastasis and recurrence

Tumor Markers

- *Associated Gene Mutations (not tumor markers)*
  - HRPT2/CDC73

Therapy

- Surgery is the mainstay of therapy for initial presentation and for recurrent or metastatic disease
  - En-bloc resection (parathyroidectomy) with ipsilateral thyroidectomy and central neck dissection (station 6)
  - Recurrence or metastatic disease are treated with palliative surgery along with calcium lowering agents
  - Medical care is limited to the control of hypercalcemia
    - Bisphosphonates
    - Calcitonin
    - Denosumab – an option for hypercalcemia that is refractory to the above options
  - Trials of chemotherapeutic agents have been generally disappointing

NOTES

THYROID CANCER

General Overview

- Most common endocrine malignancy in the United States
- 90% of thyroid nodules are benign; female predominance
- Thyroid nodules that have features that are worrisome for malignancy:
  - Solid/solitary/hard lesion(s)
  - "Cold," minimal to no uptake on radionuclide study
  - Slow growing
  - Male
  - Age > 50, or adolescence
  - Previous neck XRT
  - MEN 2a or 2b
- Most important prognostic factor – **Age**

Diagnosis

- *Diagnosis*
  - Thyroid function test – **TSH**
  - **Ultrasound**
    - Features that are worrisome for underlying malignancy
      - Heterogeneity
      - Hypoechoic
      - Microcalcifications
      - Irregular margins
      - Unorganized vascular pattern
      - Cells that are "taller than wide"
      - Lymphatic invasion
  - Indications for **FNA biopsy** of thyroid lesions:
    - Nodule *>/= 1 cm*
      - Solid, hypoechoic, with one or more of the sonographic features listed above

- Nodule >/= *1.5 cm*
  - Solid, iso- or hypoechoic, or partially cystic, with one or more of the sonographic features listed above
- Nodule >/= *2 cm*
  - Spongiform or partially cystic, without any of the sonographic features listed above
- *No FNA biopsy required*
  - Lesion less than 1 cm
  - Cystic lesions
- **Bethesda Criteria** – "best next step" based on FNA findings
  - 1: Indeterminant – Repeat FNA
  - 2: Benign – Repeat US in six to twelve months
  - 3: AUS/FLUS – Repeat FNA
  - 4: Follicular/Hurthle cell neoplasm – Lobectomy
  - 5: Suspicious malignancy – Lobectomy
  - 6: Malignancy – Lobectomy versus Total Thyroidectomy
    - *AUS/FLUS – atypia of unknown significance/follicular lesion of unknown significance

Tumor Markers

- *Associated Gene Mutations (not tumor markers)*
  - **BRAF mutation** – associated with follicular variant papillary thyroid carcinoma
  - **RET proto-oncogene** – associated with Medullary thyroid carcinoma
- Thyroglobulin (not a tumor marker) – can only be utilized to determine recurrence or metastases after total thyroidectomy
  - Stores T3 and T4 in colloid

- **CEA, Calcitonin**
  - o Associated with medullary thyroid carcinoma
  - o Prognostic marker

Therapy

- Papillary thyroid carcinoma
  - o Most common thyroid malignancy
  - o Spreads lymphatically (not prognostic, prognosis based on *local invasion*)
  - o Pathology: **psammoma bodies** and **Orphan Annie nuclei**
  - o Treatment:
    - Lobectomy
    - Indications for *Total Thyroidectomy*:
      - \> 4 cm
      - Poorly differentiated
      - Extra-thyroidal disease
      - Multi-centric
      - Previous XRT
    - Indications for *MRND*:
      - Extra-thyroidal disease
    - Indications for post-operative *Radioiodine Ablation*:
      - Tumor > 4 cm
      - Extra-thyroidal disease
      - Need total thyroidectomy for it to be effective
    - **Tall-cell variant** – very aggressive variant
      - Requires total thyroidectomy with central nodal (station 6) dissection
- Follicular thyroid carcinoma
  - o Hematogenous spread (**bone** most common) – 50% have metastatic disease at the time of presentation
  - o If FNA reveals follicular cells (*Bethesda class 4*) – need a lobectomy to determine *capsular invasion*

o Treatment:
  ▪ Lobectomy
  ▪ Indications for *Total Thyroidectomy*:
    • > 4 cm
    • Poorly differentiated
    • Extra-thyroidal disease
    • Multi-centric
    • Previous XRT
  ▪ Indications for *MRND*:
    • Extra-thyroidal disease
  ▪ Indications for post-operative *Radioiodine Ablation*:
    • Tumor > 4 cm
    • Extra-thyroidal disease
    • Need total thyroidectomy for it to be effective

• Medullary thyroid carcinoma
  o 80% are sporadic
  o Up to 20% can be associated with **RET proto-oncogene** (MEN 2a or 2b)
  o Tumor arises from **parafollicular C cells** – secrete **calcitonin**
  o Pathology – shows **amyloid** deposition
  o Treatment:
    ▪ Total thyroidectomy with central nodal (station 6) dissection
    ▪ MRND – if patient has palpable thyroid mass
    ▪ Bilateral MRND – if multifocal and/or if there is extrathyroidal disease

• Hurthle cell carcinoma
  o Most are benign
  o Often presents in older patients
  o Pathology- shows **Ashkenazi cells**
  o If FNA reveals Hurthle cells (*Bethesda class 4*) – need a lobectomy to determine *capsular invasion*
  o **Radioresistant**

- o Treatment:
  - Indications for *Total Thyroidectomy*, after diagnostic lobectomy:
    - Malignant lesion
  - MRND – for clinically positive nodes
- Anaplastic thyroid cancer
  - o Found in elderly patients with long standing goiters
  - o Most aggressive thyroid cancer
  - o Pathology – shows **vesicular appearance of nuclei**
  - o Rapidly lethal; usually beyond surgical management at diagnosis
  - o Treatment:
    - **XRT** – can improve short-term survival and improve local recurrence
    - Can perform **palliative thyroidectomy** for compressive symptoms or palliative chemo-XRT

Adjuvant Therapy

- **131 – I Radionucleotide ablation therapy**
  - o Effective for papillary and follicular thyroid cancer
  - o Not used in:
    - Children
    - Pregnancy
    - Lactating mothers
  - o Can cure bone and lung metastases
  - o Given four to six weeks after surgery (total thyroidectomy), when TSH levels are highest
  - o *Indications*:
    - Recurrent cancer
    - Tumors > 4 cm
    - Extrathyroidal disease
  - o *Side-effects*:

- Sialadenitis
- GI symptoms
- Infertility
- Bone marrow suppression
- Parathyroid dysfunction
- Leukemia
- **Thyroxine** – administered after total thyroidectomy and completion of radionucleotide ablation
  - Can help suppress TSH and slow metastatic disease

NOTES

ADRENAL TUMORS

General Overview

- <u>Adrenocortical carcinoma</u>
  - o Rare; have a bimodal age distribution (before age 5 and in the fifth decade); more common in females
  - o Half are functional tumors – present with symptoms of hormone excess
    - Cushing's syndrome
    - Virilization
    - HTN
  - o 80% present at an advanced stage
- <u>Pheochromocytoma</u>
  - o Catecholamine secreting neuroendocrine tumors that arise from the medullary chromaffin cells
  - o Rare; usually slow growing; arise from sympathetic ganglia or ectopic neural crest cells
  - o **10% rule** – 10% are malignant, bilateral, familial, in children, or extra-adrenal
    - *Extra-adrenal* – more likely to be malignant

Diagnosis/Staging

- *Diagnosis*
  - o <u>Adrenocortical carcinoma</u>
    - For the half that are functional:
      - *Cortisol excess* – low ACTH, elevated twenty-four-hour urine cortisol
      - *Aldosterone excess* – aldosterone to renin ratio > 20, low K, high Na, metabolic alkalosis, low plasma renin
      - *Sex steroid excess* – children display virilization 90% of the time

(precocious puberty in males, virilization in females); an excess of androgens/estrogens is almost always underlying cancer
- **CT scan** findings that are suggestive of adrenal carcinoma:
  - > 4–6 cm
  - Non-homogenous
  - Peripherally enhancing
  - Central area of non–enhancement/necrosis/calcification
  - > 10 HFU
  - < 60% washout
    - o If an adrenal lesion with any of the above findings is encountered incidentally (**"incidentaloma"**), the next best step is to determine if it is functional
- **MRI**
  - Will *not* lose signal intensity on opposed phase sequencing
  - Benign adrenal lesions do lose signal intensity

o <u>Pheochromocytoma</u>
- Plasma metanephrines
- Urine metanephrines and vanillylmandelic acid (VMA)
- Clonidine suppression test – tumor does not respond, persistently elevated catecholamines
  - Utilized for patients with suspected pheochromocytoma but who are normotensive
- CT scan and MRI – best test for localization

- **MRI** – benign and malignant pheochromocytomas will *not* lose signal intensity on opposed phase sequencing
  - MIBG scan – can help identify location if having trouble finding tumor
- *Staging*
  - Adrenocortical carcinoma
    - T1 – < 5 cm
    - T2 – > 5 cm
    - T3 – peri-adrenal fatty invasion
    - T4 – neighboring organ invasion
      - Stage 1 – T1, N0, M0
      - Stage 2 – T2, N0, M0
      - Stage 3 – T1-2, N1 or T3, N0, M0
      - Stage 4 – T3-4, N1 or T-any, N-any, M1

Therapy

- Adrenocortical carcinoma
  - Treatment:
    - **Open** radical adrenalectomy (take ipsilateral kidney en-bloc)
      - For Stages 1–3
      - Adequacy of resection – most important predictor of survival
- Pheochromocytoma (malignant)
  - Treatment
    - **Open** adrenalectomy
      - Ligate adrenal veins first to avoid spilling catecholamines
      - Preoperative **phenoxybenzamine** should be given
        - Alpha before beta blockade preoperatively

Neo- and Adjuvant Therapy

- Adrenocortical carcinoma
  - For patients with *low-recurrence risk*
    - Observation after surgery
    - *Low-recurrence risk* defined as
      - R0 resection
      - Ki-67 =/< 10%
  - For patients with *high-recurrence risk*
    - Adjuvant **Mitotane** (adrenolytic) without chemotherapy
    - *High-recurrence risk* defined as
      - R1 resection
      - Intraoperative tumor spillage
      - Large tumors with vascular and/or capsular invasion
      - High grade
        - Ki-67 > 10%
        - Mitotic rate > 20 per 50 HPF
  - For patients with *very-high-recurrence risk*
    - Adjuvant **Mitotane** (adrenolytic) with **Cisplatin**-based chemotherapy
    - *Very-high-recurrence risk* defined as
      - Ki-67 > 20%
      - Vena cava thrombus
- Pheochromocytoma (malignant)
  - **Metyrosine** – inhibits tyrosine hydroxylase causing decreased synthesis of catecholamines (given preoperatively or for unresectable disease)

NOTES

_____

_____

_____

_____

_____

_____

_____

_____

_____

_____

_____

_____

_____

_____

_____

_____

_____

_____

_____

_____

_____

_____

ESOPHAGEAL CARCINOMA

General Overview

- The esophagus wall differs histologically from the rest of the gastrointestinal tract in that it lacks a **serosal layer**
- Often advanced stage at the time of diagnosis
  - Early invasion of nodes; spreads quickly along submucosal lymphatic channels
- Histologically classified as Squamous Cell Cancer (SCC) or Adenocarcinoma
  - <u>Squamous cell carcinoma</u>
    - More common in Asia and Eastern Europe
    - Tobacco and ETOH strong risk factors for SCC
    - Usually upper 2/3 of esophagus
    - Lung metastases most common
  - <u>Adenocarcinoma</u>
    - More common in North America and Western Europe
    - Obesity, GERD, Barrett's esophagus are major risk factors for adenocarcinoma
    - Usually lower 1/3 of esophagus
    - Liver metastases most common
- Both subtypes are more common in men
- Symptoms: dysphagia, unintentional weight loss
- Most important prognostic factor, in patients devoid of metastatic disease − **nodal spread**

Diagnosis/Staging

- *Diagnosis*
  - Best next step for someone presenting with *dysphagia* is an **Esophagram** (swallow study)
  - **Upper endoscopy** with biopsy to establish tissue diagnosis

- o **Siewert–Stein Classification**
  - Used to classify gastroesophageal junction tumors (GEJ)
    - Type 1 – distal part of esophagus, located between 1 and 5 cm above the anatomic GEJ
    - Type 2 – cardia, within 1–2 cm below the GEJ
    - Type 3 – subcardial stomach, 2–5 cm below GEJ
- *Staging*
  - o Determining TNM staging:
    - **Bronchoscopy**, if tumor is above the carina, to determine airway involvement
    - **EUS** with FNA, for suspicious nodes
      - Helps to determine depth of invasion and to assess for the presence of lymphadenopathy
    - CT chest/abdomen/pelvis
    - PET/CT
  - o *T Stage*
    - T1a – invades lamina propria or muscularis mucosa
    - T1b – invades submucosa (important distinction because of rich submucosal lymphatic system)
    - T2 – invades muscularis propria
    - T3 – invades adventitia (no serosa)
    - T4 – invades surrounding structures
      - T4a – Resectable (invades **pleura**, **pericardium**, **diaphragm**)
      - T4b – Unresectable (invades **aorta**, **vertebrae**, **trachea**)
  - o *N Stage*
    - N1 – one to two nodes
    - N2 – three to six nodes
    - N3 – seven or more nodes

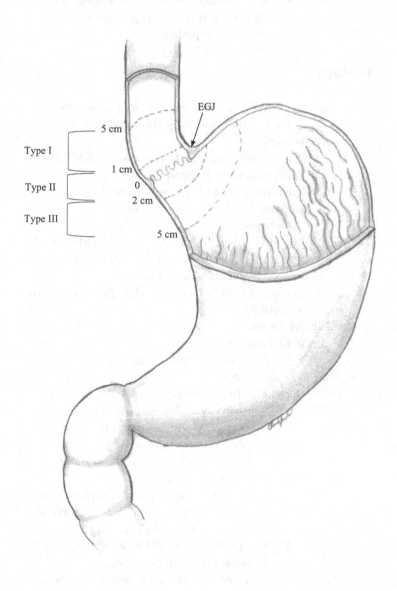

- o *M Stage*
  - ▪ M1 – distant metastases; nodes outside the area of resection (e.g., supraclavicular lymphadenopathy)

Therapy

- Barrett's HGD, in situ lesions, or T1a lesions (< 2 cm, and well- to moderately differentiated, no nodal involvement)
  - o Endoscopic mucosal resection (EMR) +/- radiofrequency ablation (RFA)
- T1b (well differentiated, low grade, no nodal involvement)
  - o Esophagectomy
- T1b (poorly differentiated, high grade, nodal involvement), T2 or greater, or any N disease
  - o Neoadjuvant chemoradiation
  - o Re-stage after neoadjuvant therapy to determine resectibility
- T4b, M disease
  - o Unresectable
    - ▪ Definitive chemoradiation
- Surgical approaches
  - o *Ivor-Lewis Esophagectomy*
    - ▪ Laparotomy and right posterolateral thoracotomy with an upper thoracic esophagogastric anastomosis
      - • Stomach serves as the conduit (neo-esophagus)
        - o **Right gastroepiploic** and right gastric arteries serve as blood supply
  - o *McKeown Esophagectomy ("3-hole esophagectomy")*
    - ▪ Laparotomy, right posterolateral thoracotomy, and a left cervical incision with a cervical anastomosis

- Stomach serves as the conduit (neo-esophagus)
    - o **Right gastroepiploic** and right gastric arteries serve as blood supply
- o *Transhiatal Esophagectomy*
    - Laparotomy and a left cervical incision with a cervical anastomosis
        - Advantages: avoid thoracotomy, leak in cervical region better tolerated than thoracic leak
        - Disadvantages: potentially smaller lymph node harvest, difficult to mobilize large upper esophageal lesions, higher leak rate
        - Stomach serves as the conduit (neo-esophagus)
            - o **Right gastroepiploic** and right gastric arteries serve as blood supply
- General Principles
    - o Approaches to esophagus by level:
        - *Cervical* – left cervical incision, along anterior border of sternocleidomastoid
        - *Mid thoracic* – right posterolateral thoracotomy
        - *Distal thoracic* – left posterolateral thoracotomy
    - o Need 6–8 cm margins
    - o Need a **pyloromyotomy** for the above procedures
    - o Conduit ideally placed in the posterior mediastinum (shorter conduit length necessary)
        - Substernal approach feasible – with greater conduit length necessary

o If stomach unavailable (e.g., previous gastric resection) to act as a conduit – *colon interposition* is an alternative
  ▪ May be first choice in young patients when you want to preserve gastric function
  ▪ Blood supply depends on the marginal vessels
o Cervical or cervicothoracic esophageal malignant lesion within (</= distance) 5 cm from the *cricopharyngeus* – definitive chemoradiation

Neo- and Adjuvant Therapy

- T1b (poorly differentiated, high grade), T2 or greater, or any N disease
  o Neoadjuvant chemoradiation
    ▪ Cisplatin and 5-FU, or Taxane based therapy + XRT
    ▪ Similar agents used for definitive and adjuvant chemotherapy
  o SCC does not need adjuvant therapy if R0 resection (regardless of nodal status)
  o Adjuvant chemotherapy for
    ▪ > T2 lesions, N disease, and/or when R0 resection was not obtained
    ▪ Nivolumab (immunotherapy) – only after preoperative chemoradiation with R0 resection and/or residual disease
      • Patient is not a candidate if they did not obtain neoadjuvant radiation therapy

NOTES

GASTRIC MALIGNANCIES

General Overview

- <u>Gastric Adenocarcinoma</u>
  - o Lauren classification
    - *Intestinal type*
    - *Diffuse type*
  - o 10% carry EBV
  - o Risk factors:
    - H. Pylori
    - Smoking
    - ETOH
    - Pernicious anemia
    - Type A blood
    - Nitrates
    - Adenomatous polyps – 15% risk of cancer
    - Intestinal metaplasia
    - **Atrophic gastritis** – Most common pre-cancerous lesion
- <u>Gastric Lymphomas</u>
  - o The stomach is most common location for extra-nodal lymphoma
  - o Usually **non-Hodgkin's lymphoma** (B cell)
  - o MALT (mucosa associated lymphoid tissue) lymphoma
    - Related to H. pylori
- <u>Gastro-intestinal stromal tumors (GIST)</u>
  - o Most common benign gastric neoplasm
    - Most common mesenchymal neoplasm in the gastrointestinal tract
  - o Arise from interstitial cells of cajal
  - o Considered malignant if:
    - > 5 cm or > 5 mitoses/50 HPF
    - Any lesion > 1 cm can behave in a malignant fashion

Diagnosis/Staging

- *Diagnosis*
  - Gastric Adenocarcinoma
    - **Upper endoscopy** with biopsy to establish tissue diagnosis
  - Gastric Lymphomas
    - Upper endoscopy with biopsy to establish tissue diagnosis
    - Laboratory evaluation (i.e., LDH, beta 2 microglobulin)
    - Bone marrow biopsy
  - Gastro-intestinal stromal tumors (GIST)
    - Upper endoscopy with biopsy to establish tissue diagnosis
    - Image guided biopsy if above unsuccessful
- *Staging*
  - Gastric Adenocarcinoma
    - Determining TNM staging:
      - **EUS** with FNA, for suspicious nodes
        - Helps to determine depth of invasion and to assess for the presence of lymphadenopathy
      - CT chest/abdomen/pelvis
        - Determines presence of absence of metastases
      - PET/CT
        - T Stage
          - T1a – invades lamina propria or muscularis mucosa
          - T1b – invades submucosa
          - T2 – invades muscularis propria

- T3 – invades subserosa
- T4 – invades through serosa or into surrounding structures
  - N Stage
    - N1 – one to two nodes
    - N2 – three to six nodes
    - N3 – seven or more nodes
  - M Stage
    - M1 – distant metastases; **Krukenberg tumor** (metastases to ovaries)
- *Staging Laparoscopy*
  - Laparoscopic staging with peritoneal washing for clinical stage > T1b tumors if chemoradiation or surgery being considered (not needed if known metastases and undergoing definitive chemoradiation or palliative options)

Tumor Markers

- *Associated Gene Mutations (not tumor markers)*
  - <u>Gastric Adenocarcinoma</u>
    - The most common genetic abnormalities:
      - p53 mutation
      - COX-2 overexpression
    - *Hereditary diffuse gastric cancer*
      - Autosomal dominant
      - Germline mutation in **CDH1** or mutated **E-cadherin** gene

- Treatment:
  - o Prophylactic total gastrectomy recommended between ages 18 and 40
- Other hereditary syndromes with increased risk of gastric cancer:
  - Lynch II Syndrome – DNA mismatch repair gene
  - Juvenile polyposis syndrome – SMAD4
  - Peutz-Jeghers syndrome
  - Familial adenomatous polyposis syndrome – APC gene
- o Gastric Lymphomas
  - t(11;18) translocation – testing should be performed in cases of MALT lymphoma
    - Presence of this translocation is associated with resistance to H. pylori eradication
- o Gastro-intestinal stromal tumors (GIST)
  - **C-KIT** positive and **CD 117** positive

Therapy

- Gastric adenocarcinoma
  - o Total versus subtotal gastrectomy is determined by location of tumor
    - 4 cm margins are required
    - Distal tumors – *Subtotal gastrectomy with gastrojejunostomy reconstruction*
    - Proximal tumors, within 1–2 cm from GEJ – *Total gastrectomy with esophagojejunostomy reconstruction*
    - At least **sixteen lymph nodes** to be harvested
      - D1 dissection = removal of peri-gastric nodes (along lesser and greater curvature)

- D2 dissection = peri-gastric nodes and nodes along the left gastric, common hepatic, celiac, and splenic artery
    - En-bloc resection of involved structures (e.g., spleen if splenic hilum is involved)
- GIST
    - o Resection with 1 cm margins
    - o No nodal dissection (hematogenous spread)
- Gastric lymphoma
    - o **Low-grade** MALT lymphoma – treat as you would H. Pylori (triple-therapy antibiotics)
    - o Non-Hodgkin's lymphoma (B cell)
        - Stages 1 and 2 – chemoradiotherapy
        - Stages 3 and 4 – chemotherapy alone
    - o The role for surgery is limited to surgical emergencies (e.g., bleeding, perforation, or obstruction)

Neo- and Adjuvant Therapy

- Gastric adenocarcinoma
    - o *Neoadjuvant Therapy*
        - T1b (poorly differentiated, high grade), T2 or greater, or any N disease
        - Neoadjuvant chemoradiation
            - Cisplatin and 5-FU, or Taxane based therapy
    - o *Adjuvant Therapy*
        - Adjuvant chemotherapy
            - 5-FU for T3-4 or node positive disease
- GIST
    - o **Imatinib** (Gleevec) – tyrosine kinase inhibitor, used for malignant tumors

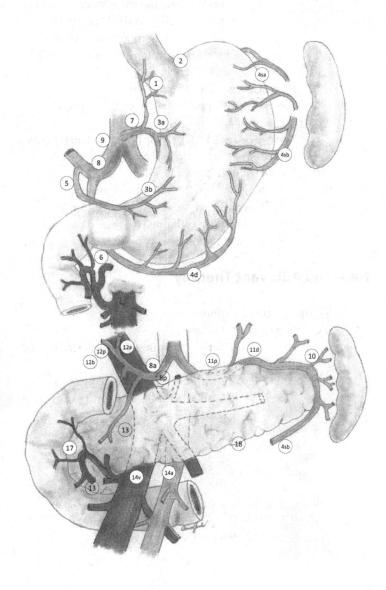

NOTES

SMALL BOWEL MALIGNANCIES

General Overview

- Carcinoid tumors
  - o Serotonin is produced by *kulchitsky cells* (enterochromaffin cells or argentaffin cells)
    - Part of amine precursor uptake decarboxylase system (*APUD*)
  - o Tumor size correlates with likelihood of metastases
  - o **Carcinoid syndrome**
    - Caused by liver metastases – liver will metabolize serotonin; therefore, patients with symptoms of carcinoid syndrome indicate metastases
    - Symptoms
      - Flushing (most common symptom)
      - Diarrhea
      - Asthma-type symptoms
      - Right heart valve lesions
- Adenocarcinoma
  - o **Most common malignant small bowel tumor**
  - o High proportion in duodenum
  - o Risk factors:
    - FAP
    - Crohn's
    - Celiac disease
    - HNPCC
    - Gardner's
    - Von Recklinghausen's
  - o Symptoms
    - Depends on site (e.g., if in duodenum can have jaundice, bleeding, or obstruction if anywhere along small bowel)

- Leiomyosarcoma
  - o Usually in jejunum and ileum; extraluminal
  - o Spreads hematogenously
  - o Cannot differentiate from leiomyoma without tissue (> 5 mitoses/50 HPF, atypia)
- Lymphoma
  - o Usually in terminal ileum
  - o Most often *NHL B cell type*
  - o Greater propensity to perforate than any other small bowel cancer

Diagnosis

- Carcinoid tumors
  - o **5-HIAA** – is a breakdown product of serotonin, can measure in urine
  - o **Chromogranin A** – highest sensitivity for detecting a carcinoid tumor
  - o *CT scan* – can identify a mass with calcifications +/- "spoke-wheel" like fibrosis of mesentery
  - o *Gallium 68-dotatate PET scan* – best for localizing tumor not seen on CT scan
- Adenocarcinoma/Leiomyosarcoma/Lymphoma
  - o *CT scan* – can identify a mass +/-
    - Signs of obstruction (i.e., air fluid level, transition point, paucity of gas in colon)
    - Lymphadenopathy
    - Metastases

Tumor Markers

- Adenocarcinoma
  - o **CEA** – elevated levels are associated with liver metastases

Therapy

- <u>Carcinoid tumors</u>
  - Resection of involved small bowel
  - Resection of involved liver – with cholecystectomy, in case of future embolization of right hepatic artery
  - Treatment of carcinoid syndrome
    - *Albuterol inhalers* – bronchospasm
    - *Phenothiazine* (alpha-blockers) – flushing
    - *Octreotide* – for serotonin mediated hypotension that is non-responsive to fluids and/or vasopressors
  - Unresectable disease
    - Chemotherapy
      - Streptozocin and 5-FU
- <u>Adenocarcinoma/Leiomyosarcoma</u>
  - Resection of involved small bowel
  - *Whipple* if involving the second portion of the duodenum
- <u>Lymphoma</u>
  - Respond very well to chemotherapy
  - May need resection of involved small bowel if obstruction is unresolving

NOTES

APPENDICEAL NEOPLASMS

General Overview

- Appendiceal Carcinoid
  - Most common tumor of the appendix
  - Tumor size correlates with likelihood of metastases and predicts lymph node involvement
- Appendiceal Adenocarcinoma (intestinal type)
  - The most common malignant tumor of the appendix
- Appendiceal Mucinous Neoplasm
  - Rare lesions – distended, mucus filled or ruptured appendix
  - Can be a benign or malignant mucinous tumor
    - **Signet ring cells** seen on histology
  - Most common cause of death – small bowel obstruction from peritoneal tumor spread

Diagnosis

- Appendiceal Carcinoid
  - The majority are found incidentally after an appendectomy
  - **Chromogranin A** – highest sensitivity for detecting a carcinoid tumor
- Appendiceal Adenocarcinoma
  - The majority are found incidentally after an appendectomy
- Appendiceal Mucinous Neoplasm
  - Appendiceal mucinous tumors are often discovered incidentally during radiologic (e.g., CT scan – well-encapsulated tubular/cystic structure in vicinity of cecum) or endoscopic workup (e.g., colonoscopy)
  - Do not perform a biopsy – risk of seeding and peritoneal spread

- o   If radiologic imaging reveals that the mucinous lesion is confined to the appendix – definitive diagnosis established after appendectomy

Tumor Markers

- • Appendiceal Mucinous Neoplasm
  - o   **CEA, CA 19-9**, and **CA-125**
    - ▪ Tumor markers are elevated in advanced appendiceal mucinous tumors
    - ▪ Tumor marker levels correlate with treatment outcomes
    - ▪ Utilized to monitor disease progression
- • Appendiceal Adenocarcinoma
  - o   **CEA**

Therapy

- • Appendiceal Carcinoid
  - o   *Appendectomy*
    - ▪ < 2 cm
    - ▪ No mesoappendiceal lymphovascular invasion
  - o   *Right hemicolectomy with lymphadenectomy* (along ileocolic and right colic arteries)
    - ▪ > 2 cm
    - ▪ Involving base
    - ▪ Mesoappendiceal lymphovascular invasion
  - o   Chemotherapy for unresectable disease
    - ▪ Streptozocin and 5-FU
- • Appendiceal Adenocarcinoma
  - o   Right hemicolectomy
- • Appendiceal Mucocele
  - o   Appendectomy
    - ▪ For benign or well-differentiated malignant lesions

o Right hemicolectomy
  - Moderately or poorly differentiated malignant lesions
  - If the base is involved and/or cannot obtain a clear margin
    - Can get pseudomyxoma peritonei with rupture, via spread of tumor implants

NOTES

COLORECTAL CANCER

General Overview

- Second leading cause of cancer death
- Symptoms:
  - Anemia
  - Constipation
  - Bleeding – blood per rectum is cancer until proven otherwise
- Association with **clostridium septicum** and **strep bovis**
- *Sigmoid colon* – most common site of primary tumor
- **Nodal status** – most important prognostic factor
- Liver – no. 1 site of metastases, no. 2 – lung
- *Mucoepidermoid* (histologic subtype) – worst prognosis

Screening

- *Polyps*
  - *Hyperplastic polyps* – most common polyp, no cancer risk (no dysplasia), usually < 5 mm
  - *Tubular adenoma* – most common (75%)
    - Generally pedunculated
    - Present in 25% of population > 50 years of age (hence, screening guidelines)
    - Carry a 5% risk of underlying cancer
  - *Villous adenoma* – most likely to produce symptoms
    - Generally sessile and larger than tubular adenomas
    - Carry a 40–50% risk of underlying cancer
    - Risk of cancer in polyps >/= 2 cm is 35–50%
  - *Serrated polyps* – have malignant potential
  - Polyps have left-sided predominance
  - Most pedunculated polyps can be removed endoscopically

- Polyps with underlying in situ lesions are adequately treated with polypectomy
- Polyps with underlying invasive carcinoma are adequately treated with polypectomy IF:
  - Can be removed in one piece (NOT piece-meal)
  - >/= 2 mm margins
  - NOT poorly differentiated
  - NO evidence of venous or lymphatic invasion
- **Haggitt Classification**
  - Describes level of invasion into malignant polyps
  - 1 – head
  - 2 – neck
  - 3 – stalk
  - 4 – base or sessile polyp
  - 5 – carcinoma in situ

- *Colonoscopy screening recommendations*
  - Asymptomatic and average risk
    - Starting at 45 years old, *every ten years*
  - **First-degree relative** with history of adenoma or colorectal cancer < 60 years old
    - Starting at 40 years old or ten years before age of earliest diagnosed, *every five years*
  - One **first-degree relative** > 60 years old or two second-degree relatives with colon cancer
    - Starting at 40 years old, *every ten years*
  - **FAP**
    - Sigmoidoscopy starting at puberty (10–12 years old), *yearly*
    - Upper endoscopy starting at 25–30 years old, *every one to two years*

- o **HNPCC** (Lynch syndrome)
  - Colonoscopy starting at 20–25 years old or ten years before age of earliest diagnosed, *every one to two years*
- o **Inflammatory bowel disease** (i.e., UC and Crohn's)
  - Starting eight to ten years after diagnosis, *every one to three years*
    - Four quadrant biopsies every 10 cm
    - For patients with pancolitis, the cancer risk is 1% per year starting ten years after diagnosis
- *Recommended surveillance interval with history of adenoma(s)*
  - o 1–2 tubular adenomas
    - *Five years*
  - o >/= 3 tubular adenomas
    - *Three years*
  - o Advanced adenomas (> 1 cm, high grade, dysplastic, serrated, villous)
    - *Three years*
  - o Hyperplastic polyps (considered average risk)
    - *Ten years*

Diagnosis/Staging

- *Diagnosis*
  - o Endoscopic biopsy for tissue diagnosis
  - o Total colonoscopy – to rule out synchronous lesions
  - o **CT chest/abdomen/pelvis** – to evaluate for metastatic disease
  - o **Rigid proctoscopy** (for rectal cancer) – to determine level of tumor from anal verge
  - o **EUS** or **Pelvic MRI** (for rectal cancer) – to determine T and N Stage
    - MRI is better at determining tumor circumferential margin (prognostic indicator)

- *Staging*
  - o TNM staging system
    - ▪ T1 – into submucosa
    - ▪ T2 – into muscularis propria
    - ▪ T3 – into subserosa or through muscularis propria
    - ▪ T4 – through serosa into free peritoneal cavity or into adjacent organs/structures
      - • N1 – 1–3 nodes
      - • N2 - >/= 4 nodes
      - • N3 – central nodes
        - o M1 – distant metastases
  - o Stage 1 – T1-2, N0, M0
  - o Stage 2 – T3-4, N0, M0
  - o Stage 3 – T-any, N-any, M0
  - o Stage 4 – T- any, N-any, M1

Tumor Markers

- *Associated Gene Mutations (not tumor markers)*
  - o **FAP** – APC gene (chromosome 5)
  - o **HNPCC** – DNA mismatch repair gene, microsatellite instability (MLH-1, MSH-2)
  - o **p53**
  - o **DCC**
  - o **K-ras** (proto-oncogene)
- **CEA**
  - o High preoperative concentrations correlate with adverse prognosis
  - o Can be an indicator of recurrence in asymptomatic patients

Therapy

- *Goals of resection:*
  - o En bloc resection (i.e., adjacent organ involvement)

- o Adequate margins
  - 5 cm proximal and distal margins for colon cancer
  - 5 cm proximal and as little as 1 cm distal margins for low rectal cancers (to avoid sphincter complex) – **LAR**
    - If there is sphincter involvement will likely need an **APR**
  - >/= 5 mm radial margins for rectal cancer ("total mesorectal excision")
- o Regional lymphadenectomy – need a minimum of **twelve lymph nodes** to be a proper oncologic procedure
- o Mesocolon – want to make sure to take the mesentery down to the base of the vascular inflow (e.g., down to the ileocolic artery for a right hemicolectomy)
- *Local excision (transanal)*
  - o An option for low rectal **T1 lesions**, devoid of high-risk features:
    - Well to moderately differentiated
    - No lymphovascular or perineural invasion
    - < 3 cm
    - < 1/3 of circumference of bowel lumen
    - No mucin production
    - Within 8 cm of anal verge
      - Up to 20% local recurrence rate for local excision, given inability to examine regional nodes
- *Stage 4 cancer*
  - o Pulmonary and hepatic metastatic lesions can be resected in conjunction with primary tumors
    - Dependent upon if patient is a surgical candidate
    - May need preoperative chemotherapy
      - Relative contraindications for resection of colorectal liver

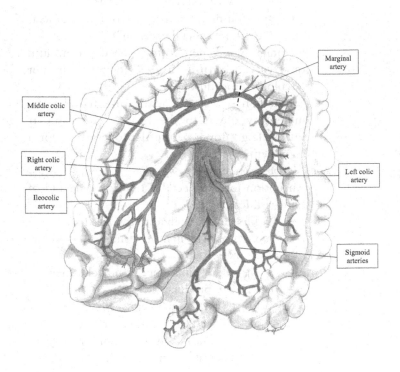

metastasis (at diagnosis without
neoadjuvant chemotherapy):
- o CEA > 200
- o Multiple hepatic metastases
- o Node-positive primary tumor
- o Bilobar metastases
- o Metastatic lesion > 5 cm
- o Unresectable metastatic lesions
  - Surgery for palliation (i.e., obstruction, bleeding, perforation)
    - Loop versus end colostomy creation for large bowel obstruction, in the context of unresectable disease

Neo- and Adjuvant Therapy

- Neoadjuvant chemo-radiotherapy (chemo-XRT)
  - o For Stages 2 and 3 rectal cancer
  - o Regimen:
    - Neoadjuvant 5,000 cGy XRT with 5-FU for five to six weeks
      - 5-FU is a radiosensitizer
- Neo/Adjuvant chemotherapy
  - o For Stages 2 and 3 rectal cancer
  - o For Stages 3 and 4 colon cancer
    - No role for XRT in colon cancer
  - o Regimen:
    - *FOLFOX* for six months, or three months preoperatively plus three months post-operatively
      - Folinic acid (Leucovorin)
      - 5-FU (Fluorouracil)
      - Oxaliplatin

Follow-up

- Follow-up **colonoscopy**
    - o At one year, to check for metachronous lesions (new primary lesions)
    - o Within six months, if total colonoscopy could not be accomplished during initial workup (to look for possible synchronous lesions)
- Endoscopy for rectal cancer (flexible sigmoidoscopy)
    - o Every three months for three years, then every six months for two years
- Post-operative CEA
    - o Every three to six months for two years
- Prognostic indicators for survival after resection of hepatic colorectal metastases
    - o Disease free interval > 12 months
    - o Tumor number < 3
    - o CEA < 200
    - o Size < 5 cm
    - o Negative nodes

NOTES

ANAL CANCER

General Overview

- **Inferior rectal artery** – supplies the anus
  - o Branch of *pudendal artery*, which arises from the *internal iliac artery*
- **Anal canal** – above dentate line
  - o Approximately 4–5 cm in length, begins proximally at the distal rectum where the mucosa blends into the *anal transition zone* epithelium, also known as the *anoderm*
    - The *anal transition zone* (a.k.a. *anoderm*) represents a region of naturally occurring intestinal metaplasia – making it particularly susceptible to HPV infection
- **Anal margin** – extends laterally from the inter-sphincteric groove to a radius of 5 cm
  - o Also known as the **perianal region**
- Subtypes:
  - o <u>Squamous cell carcinoma (SCC)</u>
    - Histologic variants:
      - Epidermoid
      - Mucoepidermoid
      - Cloacogenic
      - Basaloid
    - In-situ (non–invasive) lesions
      - **LSIL** (low-grade squamous intraepithelial lesion) – formerly known as AIN 1 (anal intraepithelial neoplasia)
      - **HSIL** (high-grade squamous intraepithelial lesion) – which now encompasses AIN 2 and 3
        - o Rate of conversion is low unless the patient is immunocompromised

- Associated with chronic HPV infection – serotypes 16 and 18
- Higher incidence amongst the immunocompromised (e.g., HIV)
  o Adenocarcinoma
    - Arise from the glandular tissue within the anal canal
  o Melanoma
    - Third most common site for melanoma
    - 1/3 have spread to mesenteric lymph nodes at time of diagnosis

Screening

- Indicated in high-risk patients
  o HIV patients
  o MSM
  o Women with cervical dysplasia
  o HPV infection – with serotypes 16 and 18
- Methods
  o HPV testing
  o Anal pap smear
  o High resolution anoscopy
- HPV vaccine
  o Recommended for individuals < 26 years old for primary prevention
    - Vaccinating individuals with underlying dysplasia is not recommended for secondary prevention

Diagnosis/Staging

- *Diagnosis*
  o Anoscopy with transanal biopsy

- *Staging*
  - o Will not need to know TNM staging, but they may ask you how to determine nodal involvement and/or distant metastases
    - Pelvic MRI or EUS +/- FNA
      - To determine T and N Stage
    - CT scan chest/abdomen/pelvis
      - To determine M Stage

Therapy

- *Anal Canal*
  - o HSIL
    - Local treatment options
      - Topical 5% imiquimod (Aldara)
      - Topical 5% 5-FU (Efudex)
      - Trichloroacetic acid
      - Ablative therapies (associated with higher recurrence rates)
      - Surgical excision
  - o Squamous cell carcinoma
    - **Nigro Protocol**
      - Chemoradiotherapy
        - o 5-FU and Mitomycin C
        - o 3,000 cGY XRT
      - Treatment response is evaluated eight to twelve weeks after completion of chemoradiotherapy
        - o A *"persistent"* lesion can be followed for six months, as long as there is no *"progressive"* disease during this follow-up
        - o Biopsy is indicated for progression of disease or persistent disease after six months following completion of the Nigro protocol

- Abdominoperineal resection (APR) for confirmed persistent (> 6 months) or progressive disease
  - Adenocarcinoma
    - **APR** for most on presentation
    - Wide local excision with 2–3 mm margins for lesions:
      - < 4 cm
      - < ½ of canal circumference
      - T1 (limited to submucosa)
      - Well differentiated
      - No lymphovascular invasion
      - No sphincter involvement
    - Post-operative chemoradiation therapy similar to rectal cancer
  - Melanoma
    - Wide local excision with lymphadenectomy
      - There is no role for sentinel lymph node biopsy for anal canal melanoma given there is no survival benefit
    - APR
      - For melanoma lesions with associated
        - Positive perirectal lymph nodes
        - Sphincter involvement
- *Anal Margin*
  - Squamous cell carcinoma
    - Wide local excision
      - For lesions < 5 cm (0.5 cm margins)
    - Chemoradiotherapy
      - 5-FU and cisplatin
      - For lesions
        - > 5 cm

- o Sphincter involvement
- o Positive lymph nodes
  - ▪ Need inguinal node dissection if clinically positive
- o <u>Melanoma</u>
  - ▪ Treat like skin melanoma

Follow-up

- <u>Squamous cell carcinoma</u> (anal canal)
  - o If there's complete clinical response after the Nigro protocol (evaluated eight to twelve weeks after completion of therapy):
    - ▪ Follow-up every three to six months for five years
      - • Digital rectal exam
      - • Anoscopy
      - • Inguinal lymph node palpation
    - ▪ CT or MRI of the chest, abdomen and pelvis with intravenous contrast annually for three years
- LSIL
  - o Observation with surveillance every four to twelve weeks
- HSIL
  - o Observation with surveillance every four to twelve weeks, regardless of which treatment option is utilized

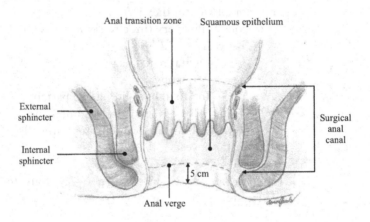

NOTES

LIVER CANCER

General Overview

- <u>Metastatic liver tumors</u>
  - The most common malignant hepatic tumors
  - Metastases tumors are significantly more common than primary malignant liver tumors
  - Metastatectomy is the only curative option for patients with colorectal liver metastases
- <u>Hepatocellular carcinoma</u> ("Hepatoma")
  - Most common cancer worldwide
  - Risk factors:
    - Hepatitis B (no. 1 cause worldwide)
    - Hepatitis C
    - ETOH
    - Hemochromatosis
    - Alpha-1-antitrypsin deficiency
    - PSC
    - Aflatoxins
    - Hepatic adenoma
    - Steroids
    - Pesticides
    - NASH
  - *Fibrolamellar type* – best prognosis, develops in adolescents and young adults
  - *Diffuse nodular type* – worst prognosis
  - Most common location for metastases – **Lung**
- <u>Hepatic Sarcoma</u>
  - "Angiosarcoma"
  - Risk factors:
    - PVC
    - Thorotrast
    - Arsenic
  - Rapidly fatal

Diagnosis

- Metastatic liver tumors
  - o **CT scan/MRI** – low attenuation lesions with mild enhancement on arterial phase
    - ▪ Focus should be placed on quantity, location, and resectability
    - ▪ Quality of liver should also be assessed
  - o Biopsies should not be performed, because of the high risk of developing needle tract metastases
- Hepatocellular Carcinoma
  - o Classic radiologic findings in conjunction with an elevated AFP are enough to make a diagnosis
    - ▪ **CT scan/MRI** – Heterogenous, poorly circumscribed mass with bright arterial enhancement with quick washout, hypodense during delayed phase
    - ▪ **AFP** – > 500 highly suggestive of HCC, correlates with tumor size
    - ▪ No role for PET/CT
    - ▪ Biopsies should not be performed, because of the high risk of developing needle tract metastases

Therapy

- Metastatic liver tumors
  - o The only curative therapeutic approach to colorectal liver metastases is the surgical resection
    - ▪ Relative contraindications for resection of colorectal liver metastasis (at diagnosis without neoadjuvant chemotherapy):
      - • CEA > 200
      - • Multiple hepatic metastases
      - • Node-positive primary tumor
      - • Bilobar metastases
      - • Metastatic lesion > 5 cm

- Hepatocellular Carcinoma
  - Few hepatic tumors are resectable at the time of presentation secondary to cirrhosis, portohepatic lymph node involvement, or metastases
  - Resection indicated for cure if solitary mass without major vascular invasion and adequate liver function
    - The necessary amount of **future liver remnant** after liver resection for cancer:
      - Healthy individuals – *20%*
      - Patients undergoing neoadjuvant chemotherapy – *30%*
      - Cirrhotic – *40%*
        - Preoperative **portal vein embolization** of diseased side if remnant is borderline (enhancing flow to non-diseased side)
    - Need **1 cm margins**
  - Patients with cirrhosis with early stage liver cancer who would not tolerate a resection could qualify for a **liver transplant**
    - Criteria used to determine candidacy for transplant (institution dependent):
      - **Milan Criteria**
        - One lesion < 5 cm
        - Three or fewer lesions, all < 3 cm
        - No vascular invasion or extra-hepatic spread
      - **UCSF Criteria**
        - One lesion < 6.5 cm
        - Three or fewer lesions, all < 4.5 cm, or a total tumor diameter < 8 cm
        - No vascular invasion or extra-hepatic spread

o **Locoregional therapies**
  ▪ For patients who are not candidates for surgical therapy, or as a bridge to transplantation
    • *Ablation* – best for small lesions < 4 cm
    • Radiofrequency, cryoablation, microwave
    • *Transarterial chemoembolization (TACE)* – for larger unresectable lesions (>/= 5 cm)
    • *External beam radiation therapy* – for unresectable lesions not amenable to TACE or ablation

NOTES

PANCREATIC CANCER

General Overview

- <u>Pancreatic Adenocarcinoma</u> (exocrine)
  - Overall, pancreatic cancer has the worst prognosis of all malignancies with a five-year survival rate of only 6%
  - Male predominance; usually sixth to seventh decade of life
  - Symptoms:
    - Unintentional weight loss (most common)
    - Painless jaundice
  - Risk factors:
    - Cigarette smoking (no. 1 risk factor)
    - Heavy ETOH use
    - Chronic pancreatitis
    - Increased BMI
    - Longstanding diabetes mellitus
- <u>Pancreatic Endocrine Tumors</u>
  - *Non-functional*
    - Represent 1/3 of pancreatic endocrine neoplasms (most common overall)
    - 90% of the nonfunctional variety are malignant
    - Tend to have an indolent and protracted course
    - Liver metastases most common
    - Most commonly in the **head of the pancreas**
  - *Functional*
    - **Insulinoma**
      - Most common functional endocrine tumor
      - Whipple's triad (symptoms):
        - Fasting hypoglycemia (< 50)

- o Symptoms of hypoglycemia (palpitations, tachycardia, diaphoresis)
  - o Relief with glucose
- 90% are benign
- Evenly distributed throughout pancreas, usually solitary

- **Gastrinoma**
  - Most common functional endocrine tumor, in context of MEN I
  - 50% malignant, 50% multiple
  - Majority found within the "gastrinoma triangle" (a.k.a. Passaro's triangle)
    - o CBD-cystic duct junction
    - o Junction of neck and body of pancreas
    - o Between second and third portion of the duodenum
  - Symptoms:
    - o Refractory or complicated PUD, diarrhea

- **Glucagonoma**
  - Majority found in the distal pancreas
  - Most malignant
  - Symptoms:
    - o Diabetes, stomatitis, dermatitis, necrolytic migratory erythema, DVT

- **VIPoma**
  - Majority found in the distal pancreas
  - Most malignant
  - Symptoms (WDHA):
    - o Watery diarrhea

- o Hypokalemia
- o Achlorhydria
- **Somatostinoma**
  - Majority found in the head of pancreas
  - Most malignant
  - Symptoms (antagonizes everything):
    - o Diabetes
    - o Gallstones
    - o Steatorrhea
- Cystic Neoplasms of the Pancreas
  - o Many encountered incidentally on imaging
  - o Most pancreatic cysts are benign, but some are pre-malignant or can harbor occult malignancy, especially if found in a patient without a history of pancreatitis
    - Pseudocyst – most common cystic lesion of the pancreas, develops after episode(s) of pancreatitis
  - o **Serous Cystadenoma**
    - Considered benign lesions without malignant potential
    - About 50% are asymptomatic and found incidentally
      - Occasionally, they can grow to a size capable of producing jaundice or GI obstruction
    - All regions of the pancreas are affected
  - o **Mucinous Cystic Neoplasm**
    - Impossible to exclude malignancy with biopsy, requires resection and extensive sampling of tumor
    - Most seen in perimenopausal women
    - 2/3 located in the body or tail of the pancreas

- o **Intraductal Papillary Mucinous Neoplasm (IPMN)**
  - Arise within the main or branch pancreatic ducts
  - Usually in their seventh to eight decade of life
  - Classification
    - Branch duct IPMN – lower risk of malignancy than MD-IPMN
    - Main duct IPMN (pancreatic duct >10mm) – higher risk of malignancy than BD-IPMN
    - Mixed duct IPMN – BD-IPMN associated with a dilated main pancreatic duct (5–10mm)
      - o Malignant potential similar to MD-IPMN
  - Management based on "Fukuoka guidelines"

Diagnosis

- *Diagnosis*
  - o <u>Pancreatic Adenocarcinoma</u>
    - Biopsy only necessary if
      - Borderline resectable lesions who need neoadjuvant therapy
      - Unresectable lesions that will need palliative therapy
    - TAP CT scan – triple-phase, pancreatic protocol
    - PET/CT used selectively if suspicion for metastasis
    - CA 19-9
    - Staging laparoscopy
      - Not universally accepted

- Some institutions suggest selective use in patients with highest probability of occult metastatic disease
  - Large primary tumors (> 3 cm)
  - CA 19-9 > 100
  - Tumors in the body and/or tail of pancreas (half of these patients will have underlying occult metastatic disease)
- Pancreatic Endocrine Tumors
  - *Non-functional*
    - TAP CT scan – triple phase, pancreatic protocol
    - Gallium 68-dotatate PET scan – more sensitive for identifying the extent of metastatic disease
  - *Functional*
    - **Insulinoma**
      - Insulin to glucose ration > 0.4, after fasting
      - Elevated C-peptide and proinsulin
      - Triple phase CT and/or MRI
      - EUS
      - NO role for octreotide scan
    - **Gastrinoma**
      - Fasting gastrin level > 1,000 pg/mL is diagnostic
      - Secretin stimulation test (>200 pg/mL), if < 1,000 pg/mL
      - Stomach basal acid output > 15 mEq/hour
      - Triple phase CT and/or MRI
      - EUS

- o Gallium 68-dotatate PET scan
- o If unable to localize with imaging, may need operative exploration
- **Glucagonoma**
  - o Glucose intolerance
  - o Fasting glucagon levels > 500 pg/mL
  - o Triple phase CT and/or MRI
  - o EUS
  - o Gallium 68-dotatate PET scan
- **VIPoma**
  - o Elevated VIP levels
  - o Triple phase CT and/or MRI
  - o EUS
  - o Gallium 68-dotatate PET scan
- **Somatostinoma**
  - o Fasting somatostatin level > 10 pg/mL
  - o Triple phase CT and/or MRI
  - o EUS
  - o Gallium 68-dotatate PET scan

- o Cystic Neoplasms of the Pancreas
  - MRCP – provides better characterization and duct anatomy
  - EUS with FNA – allows for aspiration of cyst fluid for analysis
  - **Serous Cystadenoma**
    - Radiographically – well circumscribed with characteristic central stellate scar
    - Cyst fluid – low CEA and low amylase level (benign and no communication with duct system, respectively)

- **Mucinous Cystic Neoplasm**
  - Radiographically – thick walled, single cyst with internal septations
  - Pathology will reveal a submucosa that appears like "ovarian stroma"
  - Cyst fluid – elevated CEA level and low amylase level (malignant potential and no communication with duct system, respectively)
    - Cyst fluid is viscous/mucinous
- **Intraductal Papillary Mucinous Neoplasm (IPMN)**
  - Endoscopic visualization of mucin secreting from a "fish mouth" papilla is pathognomonic of MD-IPMN
  - Cyst fluid – high CEA and high amylase level (malignant potential and has communication with duct system, respectively)

Tumor Markers

- *Associated Gene Mutations/Tumor markers*
  - Pancreatic adenocarcinoma
    - *K-ras oncogene* – 90% have this mutation
    - p53 – inactivated in up to 75% of cases
    - HER-2/neu oncogene – overexpressed
    - *DPC4 (Smad 4)* – most specific
    - p16 tumor suppressor gene mutation
    - BRCA 2
    - **CA 19-9**
      - Serum tumor marker
      - Persistently elevated levels after resection, despite negative follow-up imaging, is presumed recurrence

- o Cystic Neoplasms of the Pancreas
  - **CEA**
    - Elevated in cyst fluid indicates an elevated risk of underlying malignancy

Therapy

- Pancreatic Adenocarcinoma
  - o Tumors beyond the neck (medial to the SMV) – Distal pancreatectomy and splenectomy
  - o Tumors within the head of the pancreas – **Pancreaticoduodenectomy** ("Whipple procedure")
  - o Determining resectability
    - Resectable lesions
      - No arterial contact
      - < 180-degree contact with SMV or portal vein without vein contour irregularity
    - Borderline resectable lesions
      - Tumor contact with SMA or celiac artery < 180-degrees
      - Tumor contact with common hepatic artery only
      - Greater than 180-degree involvement of SMV or portal vein that is amenable to resection and reconstruction
      - Tumor contact with IVC
    - Unresectable lesions
      - Distant metastases
      - > 180-degree contact with SMA or celiac artery
      - Unreconstructable involvement of SMV or portal vein

- Post-op and long-term survival outcomes following R0 resection with SMV/PV resection/reconstruction are similar to R0 resection without vascular resections
- Arterial (CA/SMA) resections can be performed at high volume centers but morbidity and mortality are significantly higher
- Pancreatic Endocrine Tumors
  - *Non-functional*
    - Lesions < 2 cm can be observed with serial CT scans
    - Tumors beyond the neck (medial to the SMV) – Distal pancreatectomy and splenectomy
    - Tumors within the head of the pancreas – Pancreaticoduodenectomy ("Whipple procedure")
  - *Functional*
    - **Insulinoma**
      - < 2 cm – enucleation
      - > 2 cm and/or within 2 mm of the pancreatic duct – resection
        - Tumors beyond the neck (medial to the SMV) – Distal pancreatectomy and splenectomy
        - Tumors within the head of the pancreas – Pancreaticoduodenectomy ("Whipple procedure")
    - **Gastrinoma**
      - < 5 cm – enucleation with lymph node dissection
      - > 5 cm – resection
        - Tumors beyond the neck (medial to the SMV) – Distal

pancreatectomy and
splenectomy
- o Tumors within the
head of the pancreas –
Pancreaticoduodenectomy
("Whipple procedure")
- **Glucagonoma**
  - Resection with regional
lymphadenectomy (no enucleation
due to high-malignant potential)
- **VIPoma**
  - Resection with regional
lymphadenectomy (no enucleation
due to high-malignant potential)
    - o With a cholecystectomy
- **Somatostinoma**
  - Resection with regional
lymphadenectomy (no enucleation
due to high-malignant potential)
    - o With a cholecystectomy
- <u>Cystic Neoplasms of the Pancreas</u>
  - o **Serous Cystadenoma**
    - Resect only if symptomatic or growing on
serial imaging
      - Tumors beyond the neck (medial to
the SMV) – Distal pancreatectomy
and splenectomy
      - Tumors within the head of the
pancreas – Pancreaticoduodenectomy
("Whipple procedure")
  - o **Mucinous Cystic Neoplasms**
    - Resection indicated if >4cm or with the
presence of mural nodule(s)
      - Tumors beyond the neck (medial to
the SMV) – Distal pancreatectomy
and splenectomy

- Tumors within the head of the pancreas – Pancreaticoduodenectomy ("Whipple procedure")
- o **Intraductal Papillary Mucinous Neoplasm (IPMN)**
  - *MD-IPMN*
    - Surgical resection is recommended for all main duct and mixed type IPMNs in surgically fit patients
  - *BD-IPMN*
    - Consider resection for:
      - o High-risk stigmata:
        - Obstructive Jaundice
        - Enhancing solid nodule >5mm
        - Main duct >10mm
    - Perform EUS for "Worrisome features":
      - Pancreatitis
      - Cyst size > 3 cm
      - Thickened, enhancing cyst wall
      - Enhancing mural nodules
      - Main duct 5–9mm
      - Cyst growth rate > 5 mm over two years
      - Lymphadenopathy
      - Elevated serum CA 19-9
      - Abrupt change in duct size with distal atrophy
      - o Surgical Resection indicated if EUS confirms:
        - Mural nodule >5mm
        - Main duct involvement

- Cytology positive for high-grade dysplasia or cancer
- > 3 cm in young fit patients

Neo- and Adjuvant Therapy

- <u>Pancreatic adenocarcinoma</u>
    - o Resectable – all patients get adjuvant therapy, even after R0 resection and early stage disease
    - o Borderline resectable – Neoadjuvant therapy
        - FOLFIRINOX
            - Folinic acid (Leucovorin)
            - Fluorouracil (5-FU)
            - Irinotecan
            - Oxaliplatin
    - o Unresectable – definitive chemo-XRT
        - Gemcitabine

NOTES

GALLBLADDER CANCER

General Overview

- Rare, although the most common cancer of the biliary tract
- No. 1 risk factor – presence of stones (95% of patients with GB cancer, have underlying stones)
- **Liver** – most common site of metastases
- Larger stones (> 3 cm) are associated with tenfold increased risk of cancer
  - o The risk of cancer of the gallbladder is higher in patients with symptomatic than asymptomatic stones
- The gallbladder wall differs histologically from most of GI tract in that it lacks a **muscularis mucosa** and **submucosa**

Diagnosis/Staging

- *Diagnosis*
  - o More than half of gallbladder cancers are not diagnosed before surgery
  - o Commonly misdiagnosed as a benign gallbladder pathology, with diagnosis made after cholecystectomy and tissue diagnosis
  - o **Ultrasound**
    - Reveals a thickened irregular gallbladder wall or a mass replacing the gallbladder
    - May visualize tumor invasion of the liver, lymphadenopathy, and/or a dilated biliary tree
    - Sensitivity ranges from 70% to 100%
  - o **CT scan**
    - An important tool for staging and may identify a gallbladder mass or local invasion into adjacent viscera

- *Staging*
  - o   See below

Therapy

- The pathologic T Stage of gallbladder cancer determines the operative treatment for patients with localized cancer
- Patients without evidence of distant metastases warrant exploration for tissue diagnosis, pathologic staging, and possible curative resection
  - o **T1a** – when the tumor invades the lamina propria, usually identified incidentally after a cholecystectomy
    - *Cholecystectomy* is adequate treatment for T1a lesions
      - 100% five-year survival rate
  - o **T1b** – tumors limited to the muscular layer, usually identified incidentally after a cholecystectomy
    - *Extended cholecystectomy*
      - Cholecystectomy with resection of liver segments 4B and 5, and regional lymphadenectomy
  - o **T2** – when the tumor invades the perimuscular connective tissue without extension beyond the serosa or into the liver
    - *Extended cholecystectomy*
      - Cholecystectomy with resection of liver segments 4B and 5, and regional lymphadenectomy
  - o **T3 and T4** – tumors that grow beyond the serosa or invade the liver or other organs
    - *Cholecystectomy with extended right hepatectomy (segments 4, 5, 6, 7, and 8) with bile duct excision with Roux-en-Y biliary reconstruction*

- Only if there are no distant metastases, no peritoneal involvement, lymphadenopathy within the margins of resection

Follow-up

- Most patients with gallbladder cancer have unresectable disease at the time of diagnosis
- Recurrence after resection of gallbladder cancer occurs most commonly in the liver, the celiac or retropancreatic nodes
- The main goal of follow-up is to provide palliative care
  - o Death occurs most commonly secondary to biliary sepsis or liver failure

NOTES

CHOLANGIOCARCINOMA

General Overview

- Rare tumor arising from biliary epithelium and may occur anywhere along the biliary tree – excluding the gallbladder and Ampulla of Vater
- Symptoms
  - Early – painless jaundice
  - Late – weight loss, pruritis
- Over 95% of bile duct cancers are adenocarcinomas
- **Risk factors**:
  - *C. sinensis* infection, ulcerative colitis, choledochal cysts (15%), primary sclerosing cholangitis (10–20%), chronic bile duct infection
- <u>Intrahepatic cholangiocarcinoma</u> is treated like hepatocellular carcinoma
- <u>Extrahepatic cholangiocarcinoma</u>
  - Anatomically, they are divided into
    - Distal
    - Proximal
    - Perihilar ("Klatskin tumors")
      - About 2/3 are in the perihilar region

Diagnosis

- *Diagnosis*
  - Ultrasound – Can establish the level of obstruction and rule out the presence of bile duct stones as the cause of the obstructive jaundice
  - **CT scan** – Used to determine portal vein patency
  - PTC (percutaneous transhepatic cholangiography) – Defines the proximal extent of the tumor
  - **ERCP** – Brush biopsies and potentially for stenting for internal drainage
  - **MRCP** – Can define the anatomy and delineate the mass

Tumor Markers

- **CA 19-9** – The tumor marker, to aid in the diagnosis of cholangiocarcinoma
  - o With levels > 129 U/mL there is a sensitivity and specificity of 79% and 98%, respectively

Therapy

- Surgical excision is the only potentially curative treatment
- For unresectable *perihilar cholangiocarcinoma* a palliative biliary bypass may be performed – if not amenable to endoscopic or percutaneous stenting
  - o Unresectable tumors
    - Distant metastases
    - Lymphadenopathy outside the margins of resection
    - Vascular involvement that is not amenable to reconstruction
- For **Klatskin tumors** (perihilar tumors), **Bismuth-Corlette type 1 or 2** (CHD and CHD bifurcation, respectively) – with no signs of vascular involvement:
  - o Extrahepatic bile duct incision (i.e., common hepatic duct, common bile duct), cholecystectomy, portal lymphadenectomy, and bilateral Roux-en-Y hepaticojejunostomy
- For **KIatskin tumors** (perihilar tumors), **Bismuth-Corlette 3a or 3b** (involving the right and left hepatic duct, respectively) – with no signs of vascular involvement:
  - o Extrahepatic bile duct incision (i.e., common hepatic duct, common bile duct), cholecystectomy, portal lymphadenectomy, and bilateral Roux-en-Y hepaticojejunostomy
  - o Above procedure with right or left hepatic lobectomy, respectively

- **Proximal bile duct tumors**, when resectable, are treated like perihilar tumors (Bismuth–Corlette type 1 or 2)
- **Distal bile duct tumors** are more often resectable
  o Whipple procedure
- Patients with unresectable disease often are offered definitive chemotherapy
  o 5-FU
  o 5-FU in combination with mitomycin C and doxorubicin
  o Gemcitabine

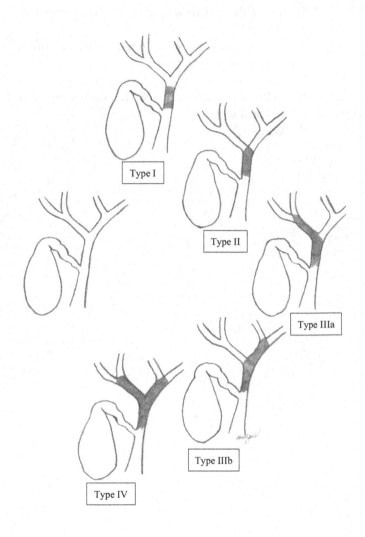

Type I

Type II

Type IIIa

Type IIIb

Type IV

NOTES

ABOUT THE AUTHOR

Aryan Meknat, M.D. completed his General Surgery residency at Brookdale University Hospital and Lehigh Valley Health Network and will be continuing his training in Cardiothoracic Surgery at Allegheny Health Network. During his final year of residency, he served as the education chief - which is when he realized there were a lack of organized and concise resources on the topic of surgical oncology, as it pertains to general surgery. He set out to compiling his notes from his five years of residency, that had served him well for the ABSITE and American Board of Surgery Qualifying Exam and created this review. His goal would be to have this book utilized as a surgical oncology resource to supplement other review books out there.

Printed in the United States
by Baker & Taylor Publisher Services